# Platform
**Papers**

Quarterly essays from Currency House          No. 8: April 2006

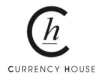

CURRENCY HOUSE

PLATFORM PAPERS
Quarterly essays from Currency House Inc.

**Editor**: Dr John Golder, j.golder@unsw.edu.au

**Currency House Inc.** is a non-profit association and resource centre advocating the role of the performing arts in public life by research, debate and publication.

Postal address: PO Box 2270, Strawberry Hills, NSW 2012, Australia

Email: info@currencyhouse.org.au      Tel: (02) 9319 4953
Website: www.currencyhouse.org.au    Fax: (02) 9319 3649

**Executive Officer**: Eamon Flack
**Editorial Board**: Katharine Brisbane AM, Dr John Golder, John McCallum, Greig Tillotson

ISBN  0 9757301 4 2
ISSN  1449-583X

Cover design by Kate Florance
Typeset in 10.5 Arrus BT
Printed by Hyde Park Press, Adelaide

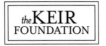

This edition of Platform Papers is supported by donations from the following: the Keir Foundation, Katharine Brisbane, Malcolm Duncan, David Marr, Tony Scotford, Alan Seymour, Greg and Fiona Quirk, Mary Vallentine and Jane Westbrook. To them and to all our supporters Currency House extends sincere gratitude.

# Contents

AVAILABILITY *Platform Papers*, quarterly essays on the
performing arts, is published every January, April, July
and October and is available through bookshops or by
subscription (for order form, see page 78).

LETTERS Currency House invites readers to submit letters of
400–1,000 words in response to the essays. Letters should
be emailed to the Editor at info@currencyhouse.org.au or
posted to Currency House at PO Box 2270, Strawberry Hills,
NSW 2012, Australia. To be considered for the next issue,
the letters must be received by 15 May 2006.

CURRENCY HOUSE For membership details, see our website
at: www.currencyhouse.org.au

# Body for Hire?

## The state of Dance in Australia

AMANDA CARD

# Author's acknowledgements

I would like to thank all the choreographers, directors, performers, writers, researchers, producers, curators, project officers and administrators working in dance and performance with whom I have discussed the general themes of this essay, over a long period. Their knowledge and generosity have helped formulate my understanding of the environments within which dance is practised, even though the opinions expressed here cannot be blamed on anyone but me. More specifically I would like to thank Katharine Brisbane for her patience and keen editor's eye and Julie-Anne Long for her direct and insightful comments as a reader. Thanks also to Maggi Phillips, Tess de Quincey, Sue Healey, Kate Champion, Jennifer McLauchlan and Josh Wright for recent clarifications, comments and challenges to the themes that I have approached here. Finally, I could not do what I do (and be so 'opinionated' while doing it) without the love and support of Beth and Robin Card, David and Finn Robbins.

# The author

AMANDA CARD spent her professional career as a dancer with Kinetic Energy, on the commercial dance circuit in Sydney, Japan and South-East Asia, and as a member of Human Veins Dance Theatre. In 1990 she traded dance for academic study receiving a BA Honours in 1994, with majors in history and women's studies from the University of Sydney. In 1999 she was awarded her PhD from the same institution. Her dissertation, 'History in Motion: dance and Australian culture 1920–1970', addressed issues of national representation, aesthetic and political influence, and sexual politics in Australian dance. Amanda has lectured at the University of Western Sydney and at Macquarie University, and has presented papers at dance, theatre, popular culture and feminist conferences throughout Australia and in the United States. She has also published articles in *Brolga*, *Journal of Australian Studies*, *RealTime*, *Journal of Australasian Music Research*, *Choreography and Dance* and the *Currency Companion to Music and Dance in Australia*.

In May 2000 Amanda joined Onextra as executive producer with responsibility for the artistic and financial direction of the company. In 2003 she joined the Department of Performance Studies at the University of Sydney where she now lectures in dance and movement studies, intercultural performance practices and social dance history. Amanda is currently the Chair of Board of Directors of Critical Path, Sydney's choreographic research and development centre, and shares her working week between the Department of Performance Studies and Onextra.

# 1
## The Choreographer, Dictator or Director?

When I was young, working as a dancer, I remember the process of creating a new work with a choreographer as predominantly dictatorial, whether I was working with a contemporary dance company, a commercial dance ensemble or in a 'tits and arse' show. The choreographer demonstrated; we replicated the movement to the best of our ability, and were corrected, concisely and consistently (if not always kindly), until the choreographer was content. The role of the dancer in my world (the late 1970s and the 1980s) was ruled by laws of replication. As dancers we didn't 'create' movement, we presented the work of the choreographer and, at best, were commended (or not) for our ability to 'interpret' what we were offered. I can remember only once being asked to come up with something entirely my own. I was working with Don Asker's Human Veins Dance Theatre in Canberra and Graeme Watson, one of Australia's great but rarely lauded choreographers, was creating *True Blue and the Dreamers* (1985). This work was set loosely around an exploration of Australian Anglo culture. The beach, drug taking and scenes in suburbia featured strongly on a set dominated by two large venetian blinds.

On two occasions during the development Graeme asked us to bring something to the choreographic table. 'Go home and return tomorrow with your interpretation of Venus', he told us one night. I returned to the studio the next day with a pillow stuffed under my sarong. Ok, a bit lame—a barefoot and pregnant Venus? On another occasion we were paired off, girl with boy, and Graeme asked us to decide whether we wanted to 'be with' our partner. We then improvised with our private intention in mind. I worked with David O'Neil, and after a short period of improvising, he began to run away from me, eventually settling into a circumnavigation of the studio. I chased him for a while but then gave up, took my sweat towel off the *barre* and began swatting him with it as he passed. The latter made it into *True Blue and the Dreamers*, as did my pregnant Venus. But I was surprised by what Graeme did with my, and others', simple responses to his provocations. The source material in most cases remained recognisable, at least to us, but dramatically transformed in the complicated passage through his process and onto the stage.

It has always amazed me what choreographers do with the material they have. And I have spent a lot of time contributing to, watching and reflecting on, what they do and how they create meaning for and with dancers and their audiences.

This paper is a reverie on that process—the

relationship between dancers, choreographers and those of us who observe what they do. It offers a view on the state of dance in contemporary Australia, both as a form of performance practice and a way of making a living. It asks questions about what is particular about the way choreographers work, examines a range of ways in which dancers dance, and how shifting trends in the former affect change in the latter (and vice-versa). It considers the relationship between a range of historical assumptions that fuel contemporary opinion and tries to offer an alternate way of looking at where we are, where we might go and how we might get there.

The questions I began with were: What do I complain about? What disturbs and alarms me about dance in contemporary Australia? And, if I ruled the world, what would I change?

There are naturally many ways that I could approach these questions, and more things than those I offer here have caused me to rant and protest. But the issues I have chosen have emerged out of a concern that, as we move into the twenty-first century, the traditional qualities of dance as an art form in Australia are not dismissed as an historical aberration or consumed by contemporary trends.

This paper is grounded within my own fascination with the act and art, the traditions and procedures of dancing and making dance. This fascination has kept me involved and makes me return, time and time again, to watch people move—in darkened halls with flexible seating, in gilded theatres under proscenium arches, in galleries, along the street, at parties, on VHS or DVD. I, like many others, believe that our ways of dancing offer us a particular way of 'being in the world'. The way we move, our experience of what we imagine our body can do, affects the way we understand and perceive our relationship with the world and those in it. It affects how we perceive space, location and time, how we relate to others and to ourselves.[1] But I do not harbour the shame that colours others' concerns about the history and practice of dancing in the Western world, or in our little corner of that world. I am not embarrassed by ballet and I am not entirely enamoured with contemporary dance or its precursors. I do not prefer Bollywood to ballroom or hip hop to highland; my subject here is the state of the art of dance in areas subsidised by taxpayers' money—the funded sector—and this means classical ballet, contemporary dance, Indigenous dance and physical theatre; all of which blend with each other, making their distinctions circumstantial, pragmatic and contested.

## Changing Practices

Over the last fifteen years dance practices and the structures under which they are practised have changed. These changes have been stimulated by historical and contemporary shifts in aesthetic principals, pedagogical preferences, and financial circumstances. Aspects of these differences and their implications were brought home to me very clearly a few years ago when I saw Byron Perry working with Kate Champion's project company, the Sydney-based Force Majeure.

I had seen Byron perform before, when he was working with another contemporary dance company, Chunky Move. This company's founder and artistic director, Gideon Obarzanek, began his work in Sydney with a group of extraordinary dancers that included Narelle Benjamin, Kathryn Dunn, and Brett Daffy. In works such as *Fast Idol* (1995) and *Bone Head* (1997) Narelle Banjamin's amazing contortions and high-voltage manoeuvres, Brett Daffy's vaudevillian characterisations and Kathryn Dunn's 'bag ladies', provided substance to the positive reputation this company was building in Sydney and took with them on their move to Melbourne in 1998. Chunky Move was enticed there by the Kennett Government's offer of significant financial support. Working out of Melbourne, audiences were again treated to the remarkable abilities of another group of dancers—Fiona Cameron, with her well-crafted, doll-like disregard in works such as *Corrupted* (1998), the beautifully androgenous Sarah Jane Howard in *Hydra* (2000), and Kirstie McCracken and Byron Perry with their incredible speed and slick articulation of just about every joint in the human body—or at least their human bodies—in many Chunky Move works.

In most cases Chunky Move dancers were not only the interpreters of their choreographer's physical language. Gideon Obarzanek's choreographic process often falls into a category referred to as task-based or task-oriented movement development. In this way of working the choreographer may ask a question, offer a statement, introduce a problematic concept in relation to an existing movement phrase or verbal statement and then ask the dancers to go away, alone or with others, and return with a physical/verbal response. The dancers show the choreographer what they have conceived and the choreographer reworks and edits the material offered in relation to the larger theme or concept of the work. It is often described as a more 'democratic' approach to the essentially collaborative engagement between choreographer and dancer.

Many choreographers have been influenced by this way of working. Meryl Tankard, Sue Healey and Michael Whaites utilise devices and procedures such as these, convinced not only by the aesthetic potential but by the efficacy of a more explicitly collaborative approach. As a result, some choreographers find themselves acting more like directors.

Kate Champion also enjoys working in this way. The contribution of her collaborators within Force Majeure, those who work in design and dramaturgy as well as the artists on stage, are explicitly referenced by Kate as integral to the development of the work the company makes. Other artists like Russell Dumas and Nanette Hassall were working with these task-based processes way back when other choreographers were still tied to a more dictatorial mode of practice.[2]

Audiences, however, do not always recognise this more democratic model. In defiance of the choreographer's assertions, they often continue to identify a dancer's movement vocabulary with the company or choreographer under which the work is made. Even open claims to a democratic practice are difficult to defend in a society that has never really come to terms with the 'death of the author'. And this despite a more-than-passing acquaintance with the tenets and application of deconstruction, cultural specificity, and a post-structuralist, post-modern sensibility. We might take for granted that contemporary artists play around with genre, deconstruct their own practice, juxtapose it with other forms, but we are still emphatically wedded to the cult of celebrity, the cult of the individual, the cult of heroic men and women. To this, for our purposes, we should add—the 'cult of the choreographer'. As such, choreographers will continue to find it difficult to extract themselves from their imposed role as the embodiment of the work their companies produce.

It is not only a celebrity culture, it's also a marketing culture. It is hard to interview a collective. It's difficult to advertise a work or a company without one name, one master mind. It can be done, as *In the Dark* (2005) illustrated, a production choreographed by Wendy Houstoun, Julie-Anne Long, Michael Whaites, Narelle Benjamin and Brian Carbee and premiered at Performance Space in Sydney. In much of the publicity for *In the Dark*, Wendy Houstoun was targeted. She was, after all, the internationally-famous foreigner in the group and responsible for the work's inception. But it made an unusual sight when nearly all the artists listed above trooped on stage to accept their recent award for Outstanding Achievement in Choreography at the 2005 Dance Awards at the Sydney Opera House. This symbolic act was made even more significant by their sharing the award with Graeme Murphy's *Grand* (2005). Two more different works you could not find. But democratic approaches to making dance can cause other problems. *In the Dark*'s award is now moving about the country and across the seas, doing time on each collaborator's mantelpiece.

Despite this example, and the disparity that exists between the working process and the public imagination, the directorial approach has come to dominate the development of new work in dance. This is not a recent development. A move toward this way of working has been gaining momentum over the last forty years. Dance writer, researcher and educator Maggi Phillips, from the Dance School at the Western Australian Academy of Performing Arts (WAAPA), has some interesting observations on this trend toward 'democratisation'. She places this move within changes emerging out of the 1960s:

> I see the [influence of a] 'directorial' approach [to choreography] actually arising from educational institutions and their strong influences from what is regarded as the US post-modern dance philosophies. If you look carefully at the statements of these practitioners, from [Yvonne] Rainer onwards, the idea of 'democracy' is a big issue and it runs side by side with the use of somatic techniques[3] that emphasise interior and very individualistic means of learning. This emerges alongside the introduction of choreography as a teachable discipline. At the same time, pedagogical theories across the board shifted to focus more and more on student-centred learning. Again focussing inwards. This is further complicated by the classification of students as 'clients' in education these days.
>
> Anyway, once you have people like Nanette Hassall,[4] who is strongly influenced by the practices and thinking of the US post-modern generations, heading dance departments in major institutions [in Australia] you have the dance world meshing in with the latest educational trends.[5]

Having identified this trend toward a more directorial manner of working, it is important to emphasise that a significant number of choreographers choose not to work in this way. Choreography, like any field of production, has its historically dominant processes and, for the moment, it is the overtly democratised that has the floor. There are those who favour a more dictatorial process, but it is rare to find a choreographer who will openly admit to that preference.

When collaborating on an article for the *Currency Companion to Australian Music and Dance*,[6] Erin Brannigan and I found many choreographers proclaiming the contribution of their dancers to the choreographic process. These choreographers ranged from the most experimental of artists to those working in more traditional areas such as classical ballet. Few artists were happy to admit a preference for being more dictatorial. Lucy Guerin was an exception. She told Brannigan back in 1997:

> ...on the one hand I am pretty controlling and when I'm making my own work the dancers don't make any of the movement—I'm pretty much dictatorial in that way, I make all the movement and the input.[7]

Some dancer/choreographers starting out today still feel the need to work in a more dictatorial fashion but sense its lack of legitimacy within the contemporary dance culture. I hope that Lucy Guerin's early comments on her process will offer them some comfort. As anyone who saw Lucy's early work, and watched her continuing success over the last few years will concur, it worked for her.

# 2
## Same, Same but Different

The title of the first work I saw by Force Majeure, *Same, Same but Different*, staged at the Drama Theatre in 2002, implied for me much more than a cryptic description of the narrative intention and content of the work. The extraordinary duet crafted by/on Roz Hervey and Shaun Parker struck me as unfamiliar. I had not seen Roz Hervey perform since her time with Lloyd Newson during the 2000 Olympics Cultural Festival in *can we afford this* (later known as *the cost of living*), or Shaun Parker since his days with Meryl Tankard's Australian Dance Theatre. Here in their duet they hardly moved from the spot—encircling, enveloping and entwining, as they responded to each other with an intimacy that could only be born out of the performers' own improvisation as they found a way to work together in response to what their choreographer/director, Kate Champion, offered them. This duet remains one of the most memorable I have ever seen.

I was also struck by a solo moment for Kirstie McCracken in the same work. I had seen Kirstie with Chunky Move, but I did not recall ever seeing her move with such exquisite vulnerability as she ascended a staircase, a feature of the striking design by Geoff Cobham.[8] When she finally reached the top, the tragic futility of her effort was underscored by a fragile satisfaction at having made it…somewhere.

Byron Perry's movement vocabulary in this first Force Majeure work was equally striking, but at times I was also struck by the familiarity I felt in watching some of the movement language he and Kirstie McCracken produced. On reflection I realised that my recognition was fuelled by my more recent acquaintance with their work for Chunky Move. The distinctiveness in some sections of *Same, Same but Different* was apparent within the context and the impetus of the work—the responsibility of the choreographer/director. But the familiarity that I felt with some of the movement language, movement I also enjoyed watching, was imbued with a different quality—one particular to these dancers, Byron Perry and Kirstie McCracken.

Some time later, in my role as producer with Onextra, I received inquiries from two choreographers wanting Byron Perry to join their new projects. Byron's reputation as an extraordinary, responsive dancer who could (and would) tackle just about anything was becoming legendary. And I remember thinking how much better off Australia would be if we had one big, well-stocked, well-heeled, contemporary dance company—a Super Group if you like. Then the dancers could stay put and the choreographers could go to them, instead of the other way around. For, as you will see, Byron Perry was not the only dancer in demand. The list below makes it obvious that many choreographers want to work with the same or similar groups of dancers. Here is a short list of some of those dancers and the companies and choreographers with whom they have worked:

# Amanda Card

| | |
|---|---|
| Craig Bary | Tasdance, Sue Healey & Dancers, ADT (Garry Stewart), Douglas Wright (New Zealand) |
| Fiona Cameron | Chunky Move, Kage Physical Theatre, Lucy Guerin Inc, Force Majeure |
| Kristina Chan | ADT (Garry Stewart), Chunky Move, Tasdance, Narelle Benjamin, Bernadette Walong |
| Shona Erskine | Sue Healey & Dancers, Lucy Guerin Inc. |
| Michelle Heaven | Balletlab, Chunky Move, Sue Healey & Dancers, Dance Works |
| Sarah Jane Howard | Meryl Tankard's ADT, Chunky Move, Douglas Wright |
| Stephanie Lake | Ballet Lab, Lucy Guerin Inc, Chunky Move |
| Lena Limenosa | ADT (Garry Stewart), Narelle Benjamin, Lucy Guerin, |
| Jo Lloyd | Dance Works, Chunky Move, Balletlab |
| Ryan Lowe | Meryl Tankard's ADT, Balletlab, Danceworks, Tasdance, Chunky Move |
| Kirstie McCracken | Chunky Move, Force Majeure, Lucy Guerin |
| Shona McInnes | Ballet Lab, Sue Healey & Dancers, Wu Lin Dance Theatre |
| Carlee Mellow | Dance Works, Ballet Lab, Chunky Move, Tracey Mitchell |
| Byron Perry | Chunky Move, Force Majeure, Balletlab, Kage Physical Theatre, DV8 Physical Theatre (UK) |

If I have left out your favourite contemporary dancer or a choreographer they have worked for, I apologise. But I hope you get my point. There is a pool of extraordinary dancers out there who are in demand from a range of local and international companies and choreographer/directors.

So what may have fuelled this apparent replication of dancers across different choreographers and companies? One reason is that these dancers offer choreographers what they need. They are experts in their field. They exhibit the high level of intelligence associated with being good at what they do, and they have an ability to be where they need to be in the short, fragmented time frames offered by project employment. These dancers are perfect employees for the small project companies and independent choreographers that dominate what is so maddeningly described as the 'small to medium sector' of contemporary dance. I say 'maddeningly' because the notion of a 'sector' invokes images of the functioning subdivision of an organised ecology.[9] What we really have, at least at the 'small' end, is a bunch of responsive scavengers who function in a state of perpetual crisis created through a life of irregular support and erratic employment histories.

# 3
## The Small to Medium Dance Company

Many contemporary artists, producers, critics, bureaucrats and market researchers blame the current trend on the passing of the 'golden age' of the small, contemporary, artistic-director-driven dance companies. I have contributed to the volume of this lament myself. Some modern or contemporary dance companies, it is true, are no longer with us—Australian Aboriginal Islander Dance Company, Australian Choreographic Ensemble, Australian Contemporary Dance Theatre, Bodenwieser Ballet, Chrissie Parrott Dance Collective, Darc Swan, Entr'acte Theatre, Fieldworks, Kinetic Energy, Human Veins (which became the Meryl Tankard Dance Theatre, then Sue Healey's Vis à Vis and is now the Australian Choreographic Centre), Margaret Barr Dance Drama Group, Paige Gordon Performance Group, and stella b.[10]

Various collectives have come and gone—Cherry Herring and ID399.

Many companies still survive—Australian Dance Theatre (founded Adelaide 1965),[11] Bangarra Dance Theatre (Sydney 1989), Dance Exchange (Sydney 1970),[12] Dance North (Townsville 1985, previously North Queensland Ballet and Dance Company 1970),

Dance Works (Melbourne 1983),[13] Expressions Dance Company (Brisbane 1985), Legs on the Wall (Sydney 1984), Stalker Theatre Company (Sydney 1989), Sydney Dance Company (Sydney 1976, previously Dance Company NSW 1969), and Tasdance (Launceston 1981).

Sydney's Onextra (formerly One Extra 1976) is one of the few companies that have changed status and survived. They became a producing organisation for dance in 1996.

New companies have emerged[14]—Balletlab (Melbourne 1998), Bone Map (Brisbane 1999), Branch Nebula (Sydney 2000), Chapel of Change (Melbourne 1994), Chunky Move (Melbourne 1995), Company in Space (Melbourne 1992), Co. (Company) Loaded (Perth 1995), de Quincey Co. (Sydney 2000), Force Majeure (Sydney 2002), Gravity Feed (Sydney 1992), Igneous Inc (Brisbane 1997), Kage Physical Theatre (Melbourne 1996), Kompany Kido (Perth 1999), Leigh Warren & Dancers (Adelaide 1993), Lucy Guerin Inc (Melbourne 2002), Omeo Dance (Paris/Sydney/Melbourne 2004),[15] Skadada (Perth 1995), Strange Fruit (Melbourne 1994), Tracks (Darwin 1994), Wu Lin Dance Theatre (Melbourne 1997).[16]

The status of some contemporary dance-in-education companies has also risen. They now compete in the same pool of funds as the companies listed above. These include Buzz Dance Theatre (Perth 1998, formerly 2 Dance (1985) 2 Dance Plus (1986)), Restless Dance Company (Adelaide 1991) and Stompin' Youth Dance Company (Launceston 1992).

Over the last forty years, out of 49 companies we have lost 15, kept 12 and gained 22. The outcome, on that front at least, seems to be not that bad. However, if we look at the changing status of some of the older companies and the structure of some of the newer ones, we can see a significant shift in the organisational structure over the last 15 years. Project-based companies dominate. Companies offering 52-week contracts for their dancers and a permanent home base are no longer the standard.

A cursory look at the financial status of these companies is also revealing. Most of the 'survivors' on our list are funded by the Australia Council's Major Performing Arts Board (MPAB) or through Key Organisations triennial funding. Sydney Dance Company and Bangarra join the Australian Ballet, the Western Australian Ballet and the Queensland Ballet under MPAB. Dance North, Expressions Dance Company, ADT, Buzz, Leigh Warren & Dancers, Chunky Move and now Lucy Guerin Inc are triennial Key Organisations. This means that they are considered significant organisations nationally and are given funding over three years. But the latter two companies, the most recent additions to the group, reveal the shifting structural status of even these organisations. Although Chunky Move and Lucy Guerin Inc have a home base, the former offers contracts of up to eight months, and the latter is a project-based entity.

All other surviving and new companies on our list are also project-based. Of the 22 'new' companies (including two theatre-in-eduction/youth companies)—21 are project-based. Add to that the ever-increasing number of artists and companies without company infrastructure that are listed in a publication like the Australia Council's *In Repertoire: a Guide to Australian Contemporary*

*Dance* (second edition: 2003), and the number of artists relying on project funding increases dramatically. In that publication alone, there are 24 smaller entities and individuals who listed themselves as having 'tour-ready' work in 2003; that makes 45 companies and individuals relying on project funding, a category which accounts for approximately 10% of the overall funding for dance available from the Federal Government through the Australia Council for the Arts.

## Project vs Program Funding

Gaining yearly Program funding from the Australia Council (a category which until recently came under Key Organisation funding) at least in dance, does not, however, ensure relief from uncertainty. A case in point is De Quincey Co.. Over the past six years this Sydney-based organisation, headed by Tess de Quincey, has 'enjoyed' an erratic and potentially fatal engagement with this Australia Council category. The company was granted Key Organisation Program funding in 2002, but not in 2003. They were back on the list in 2004 but off again in 2005.

This funding category should offer small organisations relief from the continuous merry-go-round of applications and recipients assume (rightly so) that it gives them vital support to develop a small infrastructure to sustain the company. Now, I need to be careful here. In order to avoid much 'gnashing of teeth' at the Australia Council I will reproduce the careful wording of their criteria. This yearly funding is provided to 'a limited number of significant organisations to enrich the diversity of dance practice'—a laudable goal. These grants are expressly for:

...organisations that are testing boundaries and demonstrate creative thinking and innovation in both artistic programming and administrative processes. Small dance companies and other structures that support dance practice are a priority... Applicants should demonstrate their ability to implement a program of well-planned, interconnected activities in a year, or an activity that occurs over the greater part of the year.[17]

As you can see from the words above, administrative sustainability (however 'creative' or 'innovative') is a prerequisite for favourable consideration in this category. In fact being an organisation is in itself a prerequisite, so the notion of having some kind of infrastructure is essential. But the on-again off-again treatment of De Quincey Co. by the Council has jeopardised the maintenance of the very thing the category's support had encouraged the company to develop in the first place.

Yes, yes... I hear that gnashing... There is a clause in the description of the Program grant on the same website that stipulates:

Please note that receipt of a Program Grant in one year gives no guarantee of funding or funding levels beyond that year. Each year, all applications compete on their merits for available funding.

This is the problem. What is the logic of having a grant process that commends the existence and maintenance of infrastructure, sustainability and interconnected activities over a year (and therefore encourages their development) but does not also allow for that sustainability to be sustainable? The erratic process experienced by De Quincey Co. nearly saw it go under at the beginning of 2005. It also renders life for the company's award-winning, regularly-lauded, mature director, Tess de Quincey, and the members of her company, financially and emotionally untenable. 'Until something happens to radically shift this paradigm.' states Tess, 'I am not at all sure whether a company structure is a viable model for our future.'[18]

By contrast, the experience of Lucy Guerin Inc. and Dancehouse has been completely different. Lucy Guerin's company received Program funding in 2003, 2004 and 2005, as did Dancehouse. This year both have been moved to Key Organisations triennial funding. Although I am sure that their directors and managers were frustrated by the inadequacy of the grants, this remains a good news story—one of progression to sustainability.

I agree with the Australia Council's view that not all companies can make that progression. Some must, by the law of averages, move back to Project funding. But it is a dangerous practice to move back and forth in a category seen as separate from the project-based categories that judge each round on the merit of their application. Perhaps the money from Program grants should simply be returned to Project funding—New Work preferably—or at least have the validity of the relationship between criteria, expectation and actuality reviewed.

This year De Quincey Co. is back in favour under Program grants, having been awarded another supportive reprieve from the Dance Board with a lump sum for 2006. I will watch the future of this category, and this company's relationship to it, with interest.[19]

# 4
## The Rise and Rise
## of 'Independence'

With all this evidence you could be forgiven for assuming that the rise of project-based companies and the associated project employment of dancers—the 'casualisation' of our dance force if you like—has been a generational change; an affliction of the contemporary environment. But if you talk to older dancers they will tell you that most of the small dance companies in the 1970s and 1980s did not employ their dancers on a 52-week contract either—we just didn't call these companies 'project-based'. We didn't have a word for what they were. We did not rove as much as dancers seem to do today but we were well acquainted with the disparate employment process. We all had part- time day jobs to sustain our relationship with those small companies with which we were aligned, and their choreographers.

So, it seems we may not have 'lost' a great many small dance companies over the last forty years, and the casualisation of employment may also not be new. However, what we have seen is the rise and rise of independence—the 'independent artist', the 'independent choreographer' and the 'independent dancer' who are all part of an 'independent sector'. As Sally Gardner so eloquently pointed out in 1997 at Dancers are Space Eaters at the Perth Institute of Contemporary Arts, these days such 'independence' often references the economic, rather than artistic, status of those artists who claim it. They are independent of support, as opposed to being independent of inherited forms of choreographic practice.

Many older artists lament the naming of those without a home as 'independent'. They guard their principles with a jealous zeal, principles that designate independence as innovation built on homage or rejection—one of the major tenets of Western Modernism. Typically a Modernist proclaims their independence from intimate precursors and, through a process of practical innovation, invents a 'new' practice within a particular art form. A typical, historically-sanctioned independence can be found in American dance history with Martha Graham's rejection of her former teachers, Ruth St Dennis and Ted Shawn; then Merce Cunningham doing the same to Martha; and the artists of the Judson Church returning the compliment to Merce.

Many Australian choreographers grew up in a system that served as a proxy for this type of historical lineage. A former generation went overseas, served their time offshore, and then returned to Australia bringing their new-found knowledge with them—Don Asker, Kai Tai Chan, Elizabeth Cameron Dalman, Russell Dumas, Nanette Hassall, Graham Jones, Graeme Murphy, Chrissie Parrott, Tess de Quincey, Maggi Seitsma, Meryl Tankard, Graeme Watson, and Leigh Warren to name but a few. Many in the next generation worked with them before striking out on their own—Kay Armstrong, Kate Champion, Paige Gordon, Lucy Guerin, Sue Healey, Helen Herbertson, Julie-Anne Long, Stephen Page, Shaun Parker, Trevor Patrick, Sue Peacock, Gideon

Obarzanek, Cheryl Stock, Kim Walker, Dean Walsh, Ros Warby and Michael Whaites. In the small, artistic-director-driven environment, shielded from the vagaries of project funding and the pressures of presenting work independently of company support (with a 52-week contract or not), many, but not all, of these artists made their first forays into choreography under the protective custody of an organisation—the Dance Company (NSW), ADT, Dance Exchange, Sydney Dance Company, Dance Works, Dance North, Human Veins, One Extra. Here their first works were often viewed with concessions made to their youth and inexperience.

These days emerging choreographers are generally not afforded access to the protective space of an umbrella organisation. Dancehouse, ADT and Chunky Move provide schemes that offer access to presentation processes for emerging artists. Lucy Guerin Inc has offered the same for the first time in 2005. Strut has taken the preliminary steps to assist artists in a similar way in Perth. Sydney Dance Company did initiate a few programs in an attempt to encourage the development of new work by company members, but more recently they administer the Hephzibah Tintner Fellowship in association with the Australian Ballet and the Sydney Symphony Orchestra.[20] Most of these programs, except the latter, offer in-kind support and are fuelled by the internal infrastructure of the company that initiates them. They offer a small number of emerging choreographers access to facilities and shelter from the pressures of presenting their own work out there all on their own. But there are too few of these opportunities. It may be true that there aren't fewer companies, but there are many, many more expectant graduates.

As a rule, Onextra does not work with emerging choreographers. We concentrate on development and presentation of the work of an affiliated group of mature artists based in Sydney. We minimise our reach to maximise our usefulness to a specific group of established artists. Other presenting organisations offer intermittent programs that allow choreographers to present work under their roof—Performance Space and the Perth Institute of Contemporary Art, for example. But, these days, many non-aligned emerging choreographers have no attachment to an established choreographer. They have not been party to a proxy apprenticeship—paid or unpaid. For most, their teaching institution has taken over that role.

# 5
# The Role of Institutions in the Redefinition of 'Independence'

Tertiary institutions all over the country—one or two in every state of Australia—churn out in excess of 50 graduates each year. A small minority will be absorbed into the Major Performing Arts Companies and others might make it into ADT,

Leigh Warren & Dancers, Expressions, Dance North, Bangarra or Sydney Dance Company. Some will try their luck overseas. Others find themselves competing with more experienced dancers roving the open market. The recent graduate unable to get a permanent job, or make themselves known on the project circuit, has two options—give up, or claim independent choreographic status and persuade a producer or a funding committee to offer them a chance to make work. This environment encourages graduating students to expect to be independent. Institutions have consequently become the site of de facto choreographic apprenticeship, in which the dancer is prepared for a career in which they make their own work or are employed by choreographers among whom a directorial mode of production is preferred.

In the early 1970s things were very different. Most dancers were still educated in a ballet academy. The only publicly-funded school at that time was the Australian Ballet School—a feeder for the Australian Ballet Company. Rusden College in Victoria (now Deakin University) had the first dance degree course in 1975; the Victorian College of the Arts didn't open its doors to dance until 1979. Everyone who wanted to become a dancer left school at what was then called fourth form (Year 10) aged 15 or 16 and their parents paid for two years of private tuition at a 'full-time ballet school'. Those who did not go to a private ballet college learnt to dance at institutions like Bodenwieser Studios in Sydney or the Margaret Lasica Studio in Melbourne, where you could take a variety of classes from local and visiting teachers. I caught the tail end of this era. I went to Halliday's in Sydney after leaving school at 15. Halliday's was typical of many such institutions.

We did ballet classes, fencing, acting, repertoire and 'modern' dance. In the latter category we were taught by returning dancers a generation or so older than ourselves—Graham Jones (on his way back from the Ballet Rambert in London), Nanette Hassall (when she returned by way of Merce Cunningham in New York and the companies Strider and Rambert in London), and Russell Dumas (when he returned from Strider, Rambert and Trish Brown and Twyla Tharp in the US). These dancers brought with them the techniques to which they had been exposed in Britain, Europe and America—Graham and Cunningham among them.

Today dance is a secondary-school subject in many State systems. Dancers leave school at Year 12 aged 17 or 18 and then supplement their State-funded and private dance education with tertiary dance training. These young people emerge from three or four years of advanced training at the average age of 22, clutching their academic transcript that includes units in choreography. They are older. There are more of them. And they have more expectations—like being paid properly for the work they do.

At the offices of Onextra, I get phone calls and emails from these recently-graduated dancers. They ask for advice about company auditions but, at least in Sydney, auditions seem to be a thing of the past. The directors and staff of ADT and Chunky Move occasionally pass through Sydney in search of a dancer or two, but none of the independent choreographers, those working with Onextra at least, ever have auditions. The concept seems almost antiquated. These graduates then ask how they could make contact with choreographer/directors engaged in the project-based scene in Sydney.

I answer, apologetically, that they just need to meet people where they can. Dropped into this environment these young dancers find themselves unable to compete with experienced dancers and choreographers. Many of these artists, some of whom make up our potential Super Group, push younger, less experienced dancers off the floor and back on their own devices. After all, most choreographer/directors only work with those that they know and trust. And why wouldn't this be the case? Funding structures dictate it.

## Project processes: how it all works

In dance, as in just about all other art forms, applications for funding come around three times a year. Except for the occasional special initiative, the Australia Council Dance Fund offers two application periods for projects—May and November—and Program grants are in June. Most State governments offer one application round a year. In NSW this is June for both projects and yearly funding. This duel approach requires some very strategic planning and commitment from those working in this area. It is advisable that every project-based artist or company have at least two, at best three, applications submitted in any one year to cover the next 18 months. May applications are advised in September, but a project funded in this round cannot start until October. November applications are advised the following March so projects can start in April. June applications are for the following year as well.

For those not acquainted with this process, let me complicate it for you further. Within project-based funding, discrete development stages for new work are available and encouraged. Many peer review boards in dance believe, with some justification, that a longer gestation period for a new work will make that work more reflective and effective. It is not that these organisations insist on this process but it has almost become a tradition within this sector for choreographer/directors to apply for more than one stage of development for a new work. Many have also come to value (or at least accept the validity of) this divided process. As a result, dance artists typically apply for money to make a work that will be developed over discrete periods with gaps from six to 12 months in between the stages of development.

All choreographers in all genres are acquainted with this interrupted process. Larger companies such as ADT or Bangarra may have full-time contracted positions for dancers but they also have a variety of different pressures in relation to development periods for new work. Touring obligations place restrictions on their access to longer development periods, often denying the company choreographers the luxuries that should flow from having dancers 'on tap'. For project companies and choreographers, the final stage of a new work is most likely to be four or five weeks of rehearsal, culminating in a one or two-week season and possibly, but not probably, a tour sometime in the next few years.

So, hypothetically, a project-based choreographer may decide between November 2005 and April 2006 that they would like to make a work with Bill, Betty and Bettina Bloggs. Before 15 May 2006 they will need to invent the project, secure rehearsal space, get a commitment from the Bloggs triplets and write a succinct, lucid application for a four-to-six week first stage development in the category of New Work (development only) submitted to the Dance Fund of the Australia Council. This first section of the project will not be allowed to start until October 2006.

If they choose to apply also to the State funding institution (at least in NSW) they would need to make another application in June 2006—but then the project would not start until January 2007. If this is the case, then the first stage development could take place in January or February 2007. After the first four-to-six weeks' development, the results of that first stage would be used to fuel an application for a second and possibly final stage of the work to production. For this application to New Work (production) the choreographer/director needs to not only re-secure the commitment of the Bloggs triplets but also find a lighting designer, set designer, composer, technical assistance and a commitment from a presenter. This second stage might start in October 2007 for presentation in November or December 2007. But December is a hard month to present work in Australia as is January and February. So this artist might want to wait until March, April or May 2008 to present their gem to the world.

In this all-too-typical scenario, a work that may last between 60 and 90 minutes has had an 18-month to two-year gestation. But, in the real world of the project-based artist, one of the triplets will get pregnant and another will move to Alaska or commit to a more lucrative project or more regular work. After all, the Bloggs triplets are trying to string together a semi-consistent work pattern to ensure that they eat and pay their rent. Our hypothetical employer can only offer 14 weeks' work over a two-year period. And, remember, our hypothetical scenario will only work this 'efficiently' if all four applications are successful. With the pressure on the funding dollar at both a Federal and State level it is likely this project will be strung out for another year or two.

With such large time lapses between development stages, a further hazard is keeping the original artistic impetus. First-stage developments are too-often wasted as the long wait sees an artist move on. It's a wonder there are not more casualties of the project-based dance economy, a trail of bodies expired on the road to an audience.

Of course, you don't have to do it this way. You can apply for as much as you can justify—$70,000 or $80,000 for an average project let's say—from one funding round at any one time. But, I hear experienced applicants groan. You can probably count on one hand the number of people who have been given $70,000 or more for one project in the category of New Work at one time from one funding body—in fact in the last eight rounds of the Australia Council's project funding I have counted two.[21]

There is also the option of supplementing your government funding with private money. Many artists and producers are well acquainted with the process of getting something for nothing. All beg, borrow (but rarely steal) material assistance for production and promotion from friends, family and other small organisations and companies who provide 'in kind' support for a project. But donations of cash are extremely rare at the lower end of town. I know of only one small project-based company that has recently received a small sum of money from a private donor. Organisations like the Australian Business Arts Foundation (ABaF) do their best to make the connections between business and artists, but most successes in this area go to the Major Performing Arts companies. It is a long, slow haul to encourage Australian business at the top to get involved with art practice and practitioners at the bottom. There are other options—the Myer and Ian Potter Foundations for example—but their criteria do not always fit the project at hand. This inevitably means that government funding remains the lifeblood of this sector.

So, with sources of funding so limited, the pressure to keep costs down is another powerful influence on project-based choreographers to employ proven performers, people who they know will develop, retain and perform the work effectively over time. They need to make the time in which they are together as productive as possible.

## In praise of project artists

Described in this manner, the dancers on our Super Group list, and others like them, are indeed an extraordinary bunch. A list of qualities they need and sacrifices they must make to work in this way confirms this assertion. They need to:

- have the intellectual and emotional vigour to withstand the fragmented nature of the process described above;
- have the skill to pick up and perform processes quickly and efficiently;
- be confident in their ability to create movement vocabulary;

- possess a resilient ego, resilient enough to hand over all the material they develop themselves to the choreographer/director;
- have the resources to finance their own 'down times';
- arrange their life so they can drop their 'day job' at a moment's notice;
- be happy to move regularly between cities, states and countries, in order to keep working and build a biography that will make them more employable;
- be at ease with a multiplicity of dance styles and hybrid forms of performance practice.

The same could be said for choreographers and directors. With the exception of point four, they must be prepared to do all the above but also organise, motivate and appreciate the people they work with as well as negotiate with presenters and producers, and write a damn good application to finance the project in the first place. Choreographer/director and solo performance artist Julie-Anne Long sums it up in this way:

A lot of work goes into structuring the tasks, improvisations and provocations that you use in the rehearsal room with the dancers, before rehearsals start, as well as during the process—it's an invisible effort that never ends. Constant planning and shifting continues throughout the entire process with the dancers' responses shaping the work but, for me at least, generally not affecting the direction much. I give the appearance of being easy-going and open to everything but I usually have a tight rein on where we are going. When you're in the thick of rehearsals at the end of the day the cast goes home but that's when the director or choreographer's day really kicks in. I love and hate this! I remember when my son Buster was about five months old I was committed to making a full-length work [*Body of Evidence* for One Extra (1996)]. There was so much to do to process the day and to get ready for the next day of rehearsal... I was a wreck! As a woman in a situation like that I have to say that men have the upper hand in the 'creative genius stakes'. Stravinsky's Lunch and all of that!"[22]

The identification of the relatively small pool of performers being employed by an even smaller group of choreographers and companies, will ring alarm bells for some of you. If a small group of expert dancers, our Super Group if you like, are producing a lot of the movement material for a range of choreographers who are predominantly working in a directorial mode, you might have valid reservations about the state of choreographic invention. You could be forgiven for suspecting an emerging homogeneity. After all, if everyone is abdicating responsibility to their dancers, amongst whom there is a replication across a range of choreographers, this fear would seem to be well founded.

Having said that, it is important to note that we have accepted a high level of homogeneity from a much smaller group of artists—choreographers working in some of Australia's largest artistic-director-driven Key Organisations. At the top end of town the maintenance of the artistic-director model in dance, where the artistic director is responsible for making almost all the work performed by the company, does not seem to bother anybody very much. It can't, because we keep maintaining that model, and some of those sustaining it have been entrenched in their positions for a very long time. So, if we are prepared to accept this situation, we should be grateful that so many choreographers/directors are dissipating choreographic invention across such a wide range of fabulous, intelligent sources—their dancers.

As Maggi Phillips suggested earlier, this shift has been happening for a long time, for as long as the 'democratisation' of dance has been shaping the processes by which our choreographers and dancers make work. Today with the choreographer's eye shifting even further toward framing and context, the responsibility for choreographic invention now lies more emphatically with the dancer. More and more it is the Byron Perrys and Roz Herveys who are inventing a lot of the movement language that choreographers use. It therefore seems such a shame that life for these artists should be so difficult. I know there are those who prefer it that way—the romance of the 'gypsy life of the hoofer', and all that. But it is a shame that so many great dancers find themselves so far down the food chain. Sure, a lot of them are very young—but not all of them—and wouldn't it be nice if they didn't have to always be so—young, that is. I am not saying that choreographer/ directors of larger artistic-director driven organisations are completely redundant—far from it. Only that many of the benefits they enjoy are rarely available to their project-based cousins. The erratic and itinerant work pattern of the project dancer (and choreographer/director) does not look good to the average bank manager when asking for a mortgage.

# 5
## A Dancer-Driven Model

So what about another kind of model? One that centres around the dancer? Here's an idea. We could develop more than one Super Group, one in each state and territory perhaps? In Sydney, Melbourne, Adelaide, Perth, Brisbane, Launceston, Canberra and Darwin we could make companies of between five and 15 dancers, dancers of the calibre of those listed earlier. The advantage of this model would be that these dancers would receive regular wages, regular contributions to their super funds and good sustainable working conditions—even get a mortgage if they so desired. Now wouldn't that be novel—a dancer with a mortgage *before* they retired, found an earning partner or left dance and got a 'real' job? Then, in this little schema, independent or project-based choreographer/directors could come to them. They could make works with an extraordinary group of artists and the companies could tour that work—around Australia, over to New Zealand, and then... the World!

Sounds like a weird contemporary dance company, doesn't it? But, it's not an unfamiliar model. It's how national ballet and opera companies have been working for years, but within contemporary dance circles at least, it sounds a little odd.

The notion that a contemporary dance company would employ an ensemble and have work made on that ensemble by a range of choreographers has very few historical precedents. This model has only really been an option within classical ballet. This, the argument would usually go, is due to the fact that classical ballet has no author. There is not one individual to whom the technique can trace its origin. We might blame its invention on France's Louis XIV, but it is a technique that choreographers individualise but that ultimately exists outside the individual.

Contemporary dance, by comparison, emerges from a very different historical antecedent—Modern Dance. Modern dance companies were built on the pedagogical guru model. One highly-developed individual—a rebel, a revolutionary if possible—draws together a dedicated collective. The choreographer trains these artists in their own idiosyncratic approach to the creation of movement and these dancers become the embodied realisation of that choreographer's vision. Their dancing bodies are tributes to the individuality of their choreographer's movement style. Unlike ballet, and in fact in direct response to the non-individualistic status of the classical technique, modern dance has valorised the individual.

## Ensemble companies for contemporary dance

As we have seen, many choreographers are working in a more directorial manner these days, and many are prepared to work with a range of similar dancers. So why couldn't a more 'ensemble' model work for both contemporary dancers and choreographer/ directors? Let's speculate for a second.

A scheme like this wouldn't cost much more money than is already pumped into this section of the system. Sydney Dance Company, Expressions, ADT, Dance Works, Tasdance and Buzz Dance Theatre could be turned into State ensemble companies under the direction of their current, or new, artistic directors. These new-model artistic directors would take up the mantle of that title and *direct* the company *artistically*. They could still make work themselves, occasionally, but primarily their role would be to facilitate the making of work by others. These companies would have a permanent home and reasonable facilities supported by the Australia Council and their State government's funding institution.

As Darwin and Canberra do not have local professional dance companies, perhaps the equivalent of Dance North or Leigh Warren & Dancers could move to one or other of these territory capitals. I could suggest that we lose the State ballet companies—the Western Australia Ballet and Queensland Ballet Company—but then the Australian Ballet would have to tour more, so perhaps we would need to keep one of these, but insist they collaborate with their state-funded contemporary ensembles on a regular basis. The Australian Ballet has found this productive; it has collaborated in recent years with Bangarra, offered commissions to Bernadette Walong and Meryl Tankard, developed their own dancers' choreographic talent and opened the Bodytorque series to emerging artists keen to work with the company dancers. Audiences love it.

In this schema Bangarra could remain a flagship Indigenous company in the east and we could have a second Indigenous company in another state or territory.

Imagine a contemporary dance company structure such as this, an ensemble in each state and territory, two Indigenous companies, making work by a range of contemporary choreographer/directors, presenting that work to their home audience and then touring to other cities through an exchange program and taking work overseas. Such targeted exposure would build dance audiences as we strengthened their access to, and increased their appreciation of, a range of dance forms and styles.

Such a model would not only employ a wide range of dancers and offer more graduates a place to work, it would offer project-based choreographers the opportunity to make work more regularly, be seen in larger established venues across a wider audience base both in Australia and overseas. On occasion more established choreographers could be programmed with the less established—offering developmental prospects for artists, the art form and audiences. With a range of companies and works travelling overseas, more choreographers might even be commissioned to make work with foreign companies. For, in this new regime, there could still be a range of project companies—Force Majeure, Lucy Guerin Inc., Chunky Move, de Quincey Company and others. Since our ensembles would not absorb that much more money than they already do, individuals could still make their own project work, and artists could still be assisted by an ever- expanding range of producers and presenters working in collaboration with new and established venues— a trend that seems unstoppable with organisations and state and local governments looking for inventive ways to support project artists/companies and development and presentation of new work.[23]

With access to this larger pool of choreographic talent, these ensemble companies would 'trade' on the abilities of the dancers they employ. These dancers would need to replicate the qualities of our Super Group. They would need to be extraordinary 'bodies for hire'.

# 6
# 'Body for Hire'—a Definition

The notion of a 'body for hire' is borrowed from the American dance academic Susan Leigh Foster. Foster gave this title to dancing bodies constructed through contact with many different forms of Western dance practice. In her article 'Dancing Bodies'[24] she lucidly articulates the principles and procedures that develop and maintain dancing bodies. Foster describes the way certain Western dance techniques construct dancers, and defines the principle physical manifestations that can be used to identify bodies trained in particular styles and forms of dance. Foster confines her analysis to techniques that in her estimation form the predominant 'bodies' in Western 'theatrical' dance. These are the techniques that produce the Ballet body, the Duncan body, the Graham body; the Cunningham body, the Contact body, and, finally, the 'hired' body. Foster does not include a Tap body or Jazz body, two distinctive forms of dance training, and gives no indication as to why these techniques evaded her detailed analysis.

Having said that, Foster does a great job of describing the process of becoming a dancer:

> Dancers pull, tuck, extend, lift, soften, and lengthen areas of the body throughout the duration of the technique class. They learn the curves or angles that body parts can form, and to place these in a particular shape at a given time. ... Over months and years of study, the training process repeatedly reconfigures the body. It identifies and names aspects or parts that were previously unrecognised, and it restructures the whole in terms of dynamic actions that relate the various parts.[25]

Foster also claims that someone with a vast and exclusive experience in one technique cannot transfer to another and perform its inherited movement structure without having new processes of movement imposed on their body, thus challenging, erasing, and reducing the 'imprint' of the other.

Most of the contemporary techniques she examines have an explicit or implied author:

*Duncan Technique*—created in response to the work of Isadora Duncan in the late nineteenth and early twentieth centuries in response to the strictures and excesses of classical ballet and popular dance styles of the day.

*Graham Technique*—invented by the American modernist Martha Graham in response to the pervasive nature of ballet and the lack of formal rigour in the work of Isadora Duncan and Graham's former teachers, Ruth St Dennis and Ted Shawn.

*Cunningham Technique*—created by Merce Cunningham in response to the overtly dramatic process invented by his mentor, Martha Graham. Cunningham returned exclusively to the exploration of form.

*Contact or Contact Improvisation*—developed by Steve Paxton and others in response to Cunningham's overtly-stylised form. Contact's preferred principles confronted hierarchies of ability and gender through an apparent democratisation of movement principles, locations and relationships.

*Ballet*—although it does not have an explicit author, i.e. an identifiable individual or group of individuals who created the form, the technique itself has its authority embedded in the structures and history of the form.

In Foster's schema there is one body that moves across and between the different styles of dance with no apparent allegiance to any one form or one creator. Foster calls this the 'body for hire'. This body has been formed from the desires of a new breed of what Foster identifies as 'independent choreographers'. These choreographers seek dancing bodies with numerous, but non-specific characteristics and abilities. Foster also identifies these independent choreographers as being a product of the revolutionary experiments of the 1960s and 1970s in American modern dance. At this time the very nature of what could be called dance was questioned. Many choreographers accompanied Paxton and others on an experimental journey that saw the democratisation of form, presentation and training. However, unlike their precursors, these newly 'independent' choreographers—Foster offers the American Mark Morris as an example—were not interested in developing new dance techniques that 'support[ed] their choreographic goals'. Instead they encouraged dancers to 'train in several existing techniques without adopting the aesthetic vision of any.'[26] This body:

> ...does not display its skills as a collage of discrete styles but, rather, homogenizes all styles and vo-cabularies beneath a sleek, impenetrable surface. Uncommitted to any specific aesthetic vision, it is a body for hire; it trains in order to make a living from dancing... This body, a purely physical object, can be made over into whatever look one desires.[27]

Foster does not appreciate the 'body for hire'. Where she forgives the early moderns their naive assumptions of having discovered a more 'real' or 'natural' body than those created by their predecessors, she concedes nothing to the 'body for hire'. This body, and the choreographers who employ it, cannot be forgiven their idiosyncrasies. It is less honest in its construction when compared to all other bodies constructed from other dance techniques—even ballet. It is accused of the great sin of globalisation, it 'subsumes and smooths over differences'.

The body for hire is everywhere and therefore nowhere. It has no tradition. It lacks a sense of place, a mooring to a past, a sense of tradition, location and history. Unlike the others, this body was not born from an act of revolution against an embedded enemy, or created by an individual or group of revolutionaries. This body is the ultimate capitalist body, an adaptable, globalised bricolage. With its 'rubbery flexibility coated with impervious glossiness',[28] the 'body for hire' has embraced the rotting heart of contemporary Western civilisation—popular culture... RUN TO THE HILLS!

In Foster's analysis all other dancing bodies are constructed in the classroom, but the body for hire is put together without pedagogical surveillance. The motivation for its production is purely monitory—'it trains in order to make a living from dancing.'

Foster's original identification of this 'body for hire' was described in the late 1990s, but this body—with layered training in ballet, contemporary dance, yoga, tai chi, karate and pilates—is now the primary body being developed and produced across all Western contemporary dance cultures.

Though my intention is to re-habilitate her body for hire, nevertheless I find Foster's examination of dancing bodies very useful. I like the way she analyses Western dance traditions. You could do the same for many other forms of movement. You could also look at the many different bodies constructed through certain traditions and examine the way they morph and change when they are brought to new environments like Australia. You could look at movement traditions across a range of cultures, and examine how processes of habituation make their respective 'bodies' realise a unique spatial awareness, a process of weight bearing, and ways of 'being in the world'.

I also like the way Foster restricts herself to an examination of dance practices within a Western tradition and, by proxy, validates them. Too often in our contemporary performance culture, especially over the last ten years, notions of hybridity, explorations of multi-media and the juxtaposition of different forms of art practice have been valorised at the expense of the intimate practices. Too often those who juxtapose forms of practice, trivialise the historical, intellectual and embodied conventions of dance practice in their enthusiasm for innovation.

## Innovating ourselves into oblivion

I was particularly struck by this at a recent Critical Path event where the Belgian Hans van den Broeck, a founding member of Les Ballets C de la B, showed DVDs of his most recent work, made with his own, recently-formed, company S.O.I.T.[29] At this gathering van den Broeck chatted with the audience about his work with help from Critical Path director Sophie Travers and a former dancer with Les Ballets C de la B —Australian Kathy Cogill. Hans was here as guest of Critical Path in Sydney, a site for research and development in dance, and Strut, Perth's dance presentation/advocacy/research collective, to take workshops with established and emerging choreographers—a week in each city.

I enjoyed Hans van den Broeck's work, and was struck by its indebtedness to the traditions of Dance Theatre. Here, under the turbulent skies of a Sydney night in January down at the Drill (Critical Path's new home in Rushcutters Bay—an older building being put to new use) I was reminded that unlike us, European artists and companies are not afraid of old things. They build on tradition. They do not reject the old, but repeat, expand and push within convention. It is not that they do not 'innovate', but each generation makes their 'newness' within as well as across form. They carry with them the lessons of the past and build them into new scenarios for the present; and, importantly, they find financial and audience support for doing that kind of work.

It is true that many European countries have the concentration of population to make even the most marginal of practices sustainable, but I believe we sometimes bring this lack of historical reflexivity upon ourselves. In the corridors and foyers of performance spaces I am always hearing how it's 'all been done before', if not from journalists or critics, from contemporary colleagues—others who are doing it now—or members of Australia's old guard—those who did it before. This is frustrating. Surely debate could centre around how well it has been done within the context of that form of practice.

Having used Hans van den Broeck's work as an example of exploration within tradition, I concede that his work emerges from what was originally an experimentation between forms, a juxtaposition or hybrid—Dance Theatre, which informed dance with theatre and theatre with dance. But in dance theatre (now a tradition) the work was almost always at its most profound when created from/with dancers—at least I think so. Hans van den Broeck may have started out as a psychologist when he first helped form Les Ballets C de la B but when we saw his new company's work, the bodies on display, as they jittered, jumped and jostled each other, were, recognisably, beautifully articulated dancers' bodies. They may not have been dancing. They, like all the wonderful performers in Bausch's company, or Meryl Tankard's Australian Dance, may have been skipping, screaming, signing, swinging and slapping, but they did so from an understanding of a world informed by their own embodied histories—more often than not the outcome of a serious study of the anatomical capabilities of the human body through a particular form of dancing.

That fine articulation process is not peculiar to Western dancers and dance forms. Bodies dancing, within just about all forms and techniques of dance practice, learn, as Foster suggests, to 'identify and name' (and therefore move) 'aspects and parts' of their body 'that were previously unrecognised'. Then, as they become more adept, these dancers show those articulations to us—the audience. Of course, when need be, dancers abandon these fine articulations. But even when producing ordinary movements, that ordinariness is pervaded by the potential of what that body can do. As anyone who has seen the work of Julie-Anne Long will agree, even when they blink (as Julie-Anne did for an exceptional amount of time to the strains of Mendelssohn's 'Spring Song' in *The Leisure Mistress* (2002))—that blinking is the rapid eye movement of a body thick with the traces of the techniques that have formed and informed it.

Dancers are particular. They are not circus performers (even though they might tumble and stand on each others shoulders). They are not aerialists (even though they might swing from ropes). They are not stilt walkers (even though they might walk on stilts). They are not a lot of things, but what they are, when their training has been concentrated in one technique and then juxtaposed with other dance or movement vocabularies, are beautiful 'bodies for hire', bodies capable of going to places and spaces that other bodies cannot contemplate.

## The body for hire as a state of being

Although, as I said, I find Foster's specificity useful, I want to push her body for hire out of shape. Foster, following the French post-structuralist Michel Foucault, offers her reader an overladen schema. Her dancers are always in deficit. As Foster states:

> A dancer's daily consciousness of the body... ranges between her or his perceived body—with all its pains and distortions—and images, both fantasized and real, of other bodies.[30]

For Foster our dancing body, as lived and enjoyed, seems absent. Her bodies circle around a vacuum. The overly symbolic nature of her analysis causes problems for the way dancers experience their world and their dancing. In the quotation below, her dancer's 'self' struggles to find a place to 'live':

> Aesthetic expression can result when a self uses the body as a vehicle for communicating its thoughts and feelings, or when the self merges with the body and articulates its own physical situation.[31]

In this statement we become aware of Foster's own discomfort with the development of her apparently 'subject-less' bodies. The first section offers a classical binary of 'self' and 'body'—the self 'uses' the body as a 'vehicle'. This separation pervades Foster's analysis of dancing bodies and was popular in the early days of dance analysis more generally. Later she falls prey to the disadvantages of this schema when she tries to come to grips with something that may have been fostered through her own experience of dancing. Not that I have any proof of this, of course, but I sense a disquiet which she tries to alleviate by offering that disembodied 'self' the capacity to merge with a body so that it can 'articulate its own physical situation'. I would suggest that this tension is inevitable when trying to dislocate the way we perceive the world from a location that makes that perception possible—our body.

With this dislocation in mind, her body for hire reeks with potential pathologies. Unlike their more singular, pedagogically pure cousins, the body for hire seems to be a slave to consumption, consumerism, capitalism, globalisation and mediocrity. Foster places the rise of her body for hire squarely in the 'greed is good' decade of the 1980s. This works well with her argument; this body becomes the greed-is-good dancer, gorging on a smorgasbord of styles and making Susan Leigh Foster very sick.

I concede that 'bodies for hire' are very particular bodies. They are bodies that are not manufactured purely from their sites of training. In fact, I contend that bodies for hire are not only manufactured through training but are a unique embodiment; a very precise way of 'being in the world'.

Let me tell you another story.

In 1997 I went to see the Australian Ballet perform Twyla Tharp's *In the Upper Room* (originally created nine years earlier). It was set on a vast grey stage with shaft lighting piercing through smoke and few who saw it would forget the final leap to lights out. Two women, clad in grey-and-white striped pyjamas with red sneakers on their feet, ran around the circumference of the stage—one to the right and one to the left. At full speed they met, upstage centre, ran toward us, leapt into the air, one arm up, pulled it down and landed, hitting the floor as the lights and music stopped... What a moment! After the relentless, exhilarating monotony of the Philip Glass score, the silence made you suck in air.

One section of this work is pertinent to our discussions here. Tharp had two groups in this work—the 'bomb squad' and the 'stompers', both in striped pyjamas, but the women of the bomb squad wore red point shoes and the stompers, as described earlier, had red runners. At one stage Paula Baird and Miranda Coney, two of the three stompers on the night I saw the work and the two dancers Tharp referred to as the 'china dogs', were at the back of the stage, simply running. The thing was, only one of them was *simply* running. One of these excellent dancers—Miranda Coney—ran like a ballet dancer. The other—Paula Baird—ran like a runner. Let me make my distinction clear. Of the two, Paula Baird was the one with what could be called an 'efficient' way of running. If you were a runner, her style would be the one most useful to you. Paula Baird had a way of running that looked as if she could have been a runner. She was able to replicate a way of 'being in the world', that embodied 'runner' not 'running dancer'. I know you know the difference. Whenever I have seen Paula Baird perform with the Australian Ballet I have been struck by this quality. She looked comfortable. I was always comfortable watching her. This is not comfort or safety made of complacency, or a state of watching that lacks challenge, fear, dread or expectation. This is comfort in the sense of giving yourself over, without fear, to the performer. It embodies trust. Paula always seemed to be at home in the different styles and forms of dance she was asked to perform. Not everyone in the Australian Ballet could do that. But artists like Paula Baird seem able to range across variations of form and often very different techniques.

We have all born witness to a dancer, an athlete, a singer, an actor who can range across styles and forms within, or even outside, their own practice. These performers are able to 'be', and 'become', in various and different ways with apparent ease. This is a precious gift. It may be acquired or achieved through accidents of visual, auditory and sensual particularity. It is not average, but I would also contend that it is not rare. By virtue of their adaptability these dancers are unique, as unique as those for whom one way of being/moving in the world is primary. Paula Baird was not a 'better' dancer than Miranda Coney. Miranda Coney was not a 'better' dancer than Paula Baird. They were just two distinct types of dancers. Miranda was a ballet dancer. Paula was what I would like to call a 'body for hire'.

Many critics of ballet technique believe that, taken in isolation, it can place an emphatic 'hard wiring' on bodies, often very young bodies, a wiring that is very difficult to 'decode' when offering a dancer access to another style of movement. Getting some ballet dancers to 'just run' can be a very difficult thing. However, not all bodies that find themselves at the *barre* become so exclusively inscribed. That inscription is not intrinsically a 'bad' thing even though it does produce a very particular way of 'being'. But I also think we must concede that this kind of exclusivity can only really be produced on a very specific anatomical body. On some bodies ballet technique sits perfectly. It nestles into the nooks and crannies of long lean thighs, small rotated hips, extra long arms and necks, without excessive strain. On other bodies ballet technique does not become the pervasive intruder that stifles all other ways of moving, no matter how hard the dancer tries. This can naturally cause great disappointment. There are many recalcitrant bodies harbouring the desire but not the anatomy to produce the ballet body. Such disappointment produces dysfunctional bodies, defeated psyches and zealous enemies. But is that the fault of the technique or the teaching?

With other bodies, our bodies for hire, ballet technique can become a portal to a range of skills that can be utilised to achieve certain effects. Let's face it, we wouldn't have had a Merce Cunningham or a William Forsythe without access to dancers with those facilities. (Forsythe is the former director of Ballett Frankfurt. His new company, the Forsythe Company, has just performed in the 2006 Adelaide Festival.) Twyla Tharp also revived an interest in ballet technique, the form she had studied as a child but ditched on becoming a 'serious' post-modern dancer/choreographer in the 1960s. Along with utilising other forms of dance from the popular stage, Tharp re-discovered the utility of ballet's specificity, the practical potential of 'turn out' and its relation to speed. She also re-discovered the potential of dancers who had been trained in ballet and were prepared to push it, bend it, juxtapose it with other ways of moving.

# 7
## The State of Dance in Australia

So, as we have seen, we cannot really examine the state of dance in Australia based on the premise that there has been a decline of small company structures across the country in recent years. Indeed, even more companies were created in the last 15 years than have been lost over the last 40. However, the newest of them are surviving and maintaining, sometimes by choice, a project-by-project relationship with their dancers. Added to this mix is an ever-increasing number of tertiary dance institutions producing dancers with the intention of becoming choreographers. It stands to reason that, with more dancers being trained, increasing numbers will have the ability and the desire to make work themselves. The funding institutions are aware of the burgeoning role of 'independents' in the contemporary dance ecology; they have adjusted the funding criteria and categories in all areas of project application to help manage these changes. But what they have not achieved, to date—at least at a Federal level—is significant extra funding to accommodate the increasing amount of work that could and should be made at the bottom end of town—the small end of the small-to-medium sector. The Australia Council is aware of the problems within dance in this country. They have created a regular and almost continuous stream of investigations into the 'small-to-medium sector' over the last few years, and dance has been on the receiving end of a process of replication and repetition within them—at least that is how it feels to those being asked the same questions every two years. Over the last six years we have had:

*Selling the Performing Arts* (Feb 2000)—a study of audience attendance to dance, theatre and music, which recommends strategies for expanding audiences;

*Report on an examination of the small to medium art sector* (May 2002)—which examined the viability of small-to-medium arts organisations in Australian music, theatre and dance;

*Resourcing Dance* (Feb 2004)—which looked at the subsidised dance sector and made a series of recommendations.

Guess what, there is another one on the way! In 2005, I received a visit from the charming Dr Peter Steidl, as many in our sector did. He had been commissioned by the Australia Council to develop 'a national audience development strategy for small-to-medium sized contemporary dance companies and independent dance practitioners.'[32] When he visited us at the Performance Space in Sydney all I could really suggest was that we needed more money to make more work, more regularly, so that audiences could come to small venues in any city across the country to see more dance. Work more regularly—that would develop audiences. But perhaps Dr Steidl's research interests in 'brand archetypes, consensus mapping, ingenuity and the application of cognitive science insights in marketing' will deliver a different solution—one that is possible to implement because it does not cost money—just more time and effort on the part of already stretched artists and their support teams to learn what 'consensus mapping' can do for us. I would like to encourage the Australia Council, as it moves into the first year of its new structure, to abandon its continual examination of the state of the art form. Let's not have any more enquiries into dance.

Why don't we try a new strategy? How about we just bite the bullet and get some more money from government? It sounds simplistic…because it *is* simplistic. The Australia Council's own investigative report *Resourcing Dance* bases all its recommendations, however inadequate they may be, on the 'assumption' that 'additional investment can be secured for the dance sector.'

> Given the decline in inflation-adjusted funding for non-MPAB dance in recent years, the range of issues which need to be addressed, and the lack of commercial opportunities in dance, it is question-able whether much can be achieved to strengthen the sector and build on its talents and successes without an up lift in funding.[33]

The report recommends that between $3million and $5million be secured from government sources for dance. I like Robin Archer's idea more—the same amount of money for the bottom end of town as is given to the top.[34]

In an attempt not simply to criticise the funding institutions, we could claim that the current moment offers us a window of opportunity. We have a new Australia Council structure of management and therefore the potential for change is rife. There are new, art-form-based directorial positions whose stated job description includes a responsibility to 'set strategic priorities for their art forms'.[35] On another section of the web site it is claimed that these art-form directors will have a role in 'setting strategic priorities for the entire Council and in representing their art form area across all areas of Australia Council activity'. Does that include lobbying government for more money? Or at least lobbying those with influence who will lobby government for more money, especially for the bottom ten per cent—the project-based individual artists and companies in dance? After all, in the project-based sector, as Keith Gallasch reminded us, we have some of the most adaptable dance artists, both in their development of form and their ability to survive.[36] (But it would be nice if they had access to more than 10% of the available funds on which to adapt and survive.)

We also have a new set of relationships. The new director of each art form—Dance, Literature, Music, Theatre, Visual Arts & Craft—is linked to the directors of Key Organisations, Major Performing Arts, Community Partnerships/Market Development.[37] The development of these new relationships could produce some useful dialogue, debate and action. With each art-form director working in collaboration with the director of Key Organisations and Major Performing Arts we hope that some real changes can be made in the latter sectors of the dance 'ecology', sectors that suck in so much money and, in some cases, produce so little for so many.

The Key Organisations section is modelled on the Major Performing Arts Board and will be organised into art-form 'clusters', but funding decisions will still be made by the art-form boards. One of the most interesting objectives of this section is its undertaking to 'provide operational and planning advice to key organisations, assisting companies in transition, including those moving into, or possibly out of, ongoing commitments from the Australia Council'. Between the new Director of Dance and the staff of Key Organisations and the Major Performing Arts sections of the Australia Council, I hope some fine and feisty discussions will be had in regard to the historical maintenance of their sectors. I wish them well as together they prise open the Major Performing Arts companies and the Key Organisations triennial funds for dance and have a good hard look at how that money is spent.

I have high hopes for (read expectations of) our new arrival, the new Director of Dance—Ms Jennifer McLauchlan, who comes from Britain. What is heartening about her appointment is that she therefore comes from a place where over a number of years dance has risen in status to the point where it is now seen as leading the way among the performing arts with larger audiences, making more work of higher quality and with a burgeoning cross-cultural exploration of form and content. The fact that this was achieved through a lottery system that poured money into the development and production of art and arts presentation does, however, do nothing to weaken our continued calls for more money to be directed toward dance in this country. Perhaps Ms McLauchlin will be so incredulous at the position of dance here—our lower-class status when compared to the other art forms—that she will rattle some cages and make some changes and avoid being institutionalised into the same complacency that pervades some areas of the art form she has come here to represent.

Together, at this moment when the dancing nation holds its collective breath, our new Australia Council directors could join together to challenge the historical complacency, parochial pressure, and mutating mediocrity in dance that has inflicted the top end of town for so long. The criteria against which these companies are funded needs an overhaul. The expectations of best practice, innovation (within form), and risk-taking need to be applied to all dance companies, not a few project-based companies and choreographers that scratch together a living at the bottom. We need to reinvigorate dance in Australia—for the sake of excellence of the form, the health and well-being of our creative artists, and for the attention and attraction of audiences. We need a new system—an alternate way of employing choreographers and a new deal for dancers.

Perhaps our ensembles, our Super Groups, are the answer? Not only would they offer dancers and project-based choreographers more regular and sustained employment, but this model would also go some way toward relieving our artistic directors of the great millstones they have hung around their necks when they take up the mantle. Under pressure to produce new works regularly over inordinate amounts of time without access to regular sabbatical, stifles, stagnates and stymies the very thing that placed many of these artists in their position in the first place—their creative capacities.

Our contemporary generation of choreographer/directors have been more savvy than their precursors. Artistic directors like Garry Stewart and Gideon Obarzanek and, on a smaller scale, Lucy Guerin and Kate Champion have been able to structure their worlds in a manner that allows them to diversify and avoid some of the most crippling restrictions that artistic direction has to offer. The ensemble might not be a panacea, but it does offer a way of avoiding one of the great horrors of the guru model of contemporary artistic-director dance companies of the past—the mediocrity of monotony.

In a recent article, Hilary Crampton wrote: 'Australia's grass-roots dance scene is being starved.'[38] The subject matter was primarily the Melbourne project-based dance scene and I had thought that Melbourne was the exception to the rule. Instead she highlights how impossible it is for artists to 'develop their artistry and a public profile' when they can only present work 'intermittently on a tiny scale'. I could not agree more. In the same article she also warns, 'if we do not nurture artists at this level to their fullest creative capabilities, what future do our larger organisations have?' Indeed. So, if she is to be believed, then it is 'bad all over' at the bottom end of (every) town in Australian dance these days.

So I offer this paper to those of you who do not know dance well, in the hope that you may learn more about it, be intrigued by its particularity, be incensed by its lack of status and the lack of money at its 'engine room' of choreographic practice. And I offer this to those of you who 'know' dance, as a provocation for debate at a moment of change where we could make a difference.

# Endnotes

1. This understanding of the world is drawn from the philosophical tenets of phenomenology. In particular the work of Maurice Merleau-Ponty has resonance for dancers and choreographers. See Dermot Moran, *Introduction to Phenomenology* (London: Routledge 2000) and Maurice Merleau-Ponty, *The Primacy of Perception* (Illinois: Northwestern University Press 1964).

2. See Elizabeth Dempster (ed.), *Russell Dumas, case study* (Melbourne: Deakin University Press 1990).

3. Somatic techniques collectively describe movement-training methods such as the Alexander Technique, the Feldenkrais Method, Ideokinesis, Body-Mind Centering and Release Technique. These forms of training are used by teachers, dancers and choreographers to contest and/or support other forms of dance training.

4. Nanette Hassall is currently the Director of Dance at the West Australian Academy of the Performing Arts (WAAPA).

5. Personal correspondence with Maggi Phillips, November 2005.

6. Erin Brannigan and Amanda Card, 'Choreography', in gen. eds John Whiteoak and Aline Scott-Maxwell *Currency Companion to Music and Dance in Australia* (Sydney: Currency House 2003).

7. Erin Brannigan interview with Lucy Guerin, July 1997.

8. Both Geoff Cobham and Roz Hervey are listed as Force

Majeure's associate directors with Kate Champion as artistic director: www.forcemajeure.com.au.

9    Keith Gallasch used this ecological metaphor to great effect is his own *Platform Paper*. He attributes the naming of dance as an ecosystem to me but the first time I can recall this metaphor used to describe the functioning of the dance field was during a presentation by Shirley McKechnie at Green Mill 1997 in Melbourne.

10   Rosalind Crisp's company stella b. is a special case. Although this company no longer exists, Rosalind has turned her Sydney-based Omeo Dance, originally a studio for the development and dissemination of her practice, into an association—Omeo Dance Association, based in France and Australia—as well as the related entity, Company Rosalind Crisp, under which she performs her solo work and collaborations devised and performed across Europe and in Australia.

11   Dates designate the year the organisation was formed. Information from company websites and the National Library's Australia Dancing – www.australiadancing. org.au.

12   Dance Exchange is still operational, but this company has downsized their Australian operations in the last few years due to lack of funding.

13   Although Dance Works is included here, their recent loss of Australia Council Key Organisation support may jeopardise this company's 'survival' status in the near future; a shame for such a long-standing company with such a great history.

14   'New' is defined here as any company created after 1990 that still exists. This is an arbitrary distinction, one used for convenience. Bangarra, Company in Space, Gravity Feed fall on the cusp of this period and could have made it into another category. This distinction does not apply to the companies listed as

no longer in existence; some on this list were created in the 1940s and 1950s, others more recently.

15 See note 10 for details

16 Some of the listings that I have made here will be contentious for some, especially in light of later claims I make in regard to what dance is, and is not. However, those companies that do not strictly fit the 'contemporary' dance category have many artists working within them who consider what they do to be *contemporary* dance. Particularly contentious will be the inclusion of some physical theatre/circus-based companies and the exclusion of many traditional Indigenous dance companies and other professional and semi-professional companies that work in traditional dance forms derived from other cultures. But then, I had to draw the line somewhere, so I did.

17 Australia Council website www.ozco.gov.au/grants/grants_dance/program_2006

18 Personal correspondence with Tess de Quincey, Feb 2005

19 Other organisations, like Russell Dumas's Dance Exchange, are able to tell a similar story.

20 The latest fellowship was awarded to Narelle Benjamin. She has made a film with dancers from Sydney Dance Company and will make a new live work for both Sydney Dance Company and the Australian Ballet in 2006. Her first two live works, *Inside Out* (2003) and *Out of Water* (2005), were made with Onextra, financed by the NSW Ministry of the Arts and presented at the Performance Space in Sydney. This is a rare example of the struggle at the bottom end of town eventually paying off at the top, but with no direct assistance from Federal funds on the way.

21 Australia Council Grant Round Assessment Papers 2002–2005.

22  Personal correspondence with Julie-Anne Long, February 2006. Julie-Anne's latest choreographer/director role was acknowledged at the recent Australian Dance Awards where *The Nun's Picnic* (2004) received the award for Outstanding Achievement in Independent Dance.

23  One of the biggest developments in supporting this shift are the venue-based producing units for contemporary art practice that are springing up all over the country. In Sydney the closing of Performance Space and the opening of a new contemporary arts precinct—the Carriage Works in Redfern (due 2007), supported by the NSW Government—will dramatically change the landscape for development and presentation of contemporary performance/art, including dance, in this city. In Melbourne the convening of the Arts House consortium of venues—North Melbourne Town Hall, the Meat Works and Horti Hall, supported by the Melbourne City Council—has begun to do the same. The spread of these venue-based/producer-led models has the potential to offer project-based dance artists more support for the development and presentation of new work in these cities. Perth has had its own Institute for Contemporary Arts (PICA) for many years and Brisbane's Powerhouse was also a city-based initiative at its inception. These organisations are, of course, not a complete solution to all the ills that plague project-based dance artists. They provide presentation assistance, which is vital, but the need for day-to-day administrative support—the kind that Onextra has been providing in Sydney and Strut is beginning to develop in Perth—is still a major need for small, project-based companies and individual choreographer/directors across Australia. These new venue-based presenting organisations need to take this into account, otherwise

they will have no project-based organisations and/or individuals to deal with—the pressures of 'doing it all' will continue to take its toll and more and more experienced, project-based choreographer/directors will be forced to move on.

24  Susan Leigh Foster, 'Dancing Bodies', in ed. Jane C. Desmond, *Meaning in Motion: New Cultural Studies in Dance* (Durham: Durham University Press 1997)

25  Foster, 253.

26  Foster, 255.

27  Foster, 255.

28  Foster, 255.

29  S.O.I.T. = Stay Only If Temporary.

30  Foster, 241.

31  Foster, 241.

32  From Dr Peter Steidl's biography which appeared in 'Why are we all spending money on the arts?' *Arts Hub Australia*, 10 October 2005, www.artshub.com.au.

33  *Resourcing Dance: an analysis of the subsidised Australian Dance Sector*, Australia Council, 2004, p. 63.

34  Robin Archer, 'Myth of the Mainstream', *Platform Papers*, No 4 (Sydney: Currency House April 2005).

35  *Planning for the Future: Updated Implementation Strategy*, Australia Council, 2005, p. 6.

36  Gallasch, 18–21.

37  *Planning for the Future: Implementation Strategy*, Australia Council, 2005, p. 5 Aboriginal and Torres Strait Islander Arts (ATSIA) is a separate division. There is a dotted line on the graph between the new art form directors and ATSIA which I presume denotes consultation but of a less concrete kind.

38  Hilary Crampton, 'Australia's grass-roots dance scene is being starved', *Age*, 6 January 2006.

# Contributors

David Adair, Sue Fisher and Susan Kukucka are members of Sustaining Culture, a joint research project on the role of Australia's major performing arts centres.
www.griffith.edu.au/centre/cpci/sustainigncultures/hom.html

Catherine Baldwin is chief executive of the Institute of Actuaries of Australia.

Andrew Barnum is program director of communication design at the Billy Blue School of Graphic Arts, and a visual identity lecturer at the University of Technology, Sydney (UTS).

Gillian McCracken is a freelance curator and writer.

Benjamin Marks is an Austrian school economist.

Raymond Menmuir is a producer/director.

Dr Mark Seton is associate lecturer in Performance Studies at Macquarie University.

# Readers' Forum

Such has been the response to David Throsby's *Platform Papers* 7, 'Does Australia Need a Cultural Policy?' that we are able to publish here only extracts from seven letters. We hope to take up the issue again in our next edition.

## David Adair, Sue Fisher and Susan Kukucka on sustaining culture

David Throsby's 'Does Australia Need a Cultural Policy?' is a timely contribution, highlighting the inadequacy of current approaches to valuing culture. He argues that there is a danger in being overly reliant on describing the value of culture in economic terms and as such we fail to capture the true range of values. For Throsby there are clear links between this trend and the current political climate.

In recent years the absence of an appreciation of multiple values has resulted in emphasis on social and economic imperatives. There have been many studies of the health benefits of arts participation and the role of the arts in facilitating educational attainment. Other studies have focused on economic impacts: the flow-on effects of the arts, the sector's size, and its contribution to cultural tourism. Yet while business and government have developed a language of 'performance indicators', these are able to communicate direct quantitative outcomes more easily than to describe the contexts of cultural practices and to measure their intrinsic values.

Griffith University is undertaking an Australian Research Council-funded study of Australia's flagship performing arts centres. *Sustaining Culture: the Role of Performing Arts Centres* sees Griffith University collaborating with Sydney Opera House, Queensland Performing Arts Centre, Adelaide Festival Centre, and the Arts Centre, Melbourne to produce innovative research and rigorous data that describes a centre's social, cultural, environmental, educational and economic values and impacts. It also sets out to develop ways of measuring these values, and propose a more effective language to convey these values to the public. The ability to grasp the array of current and potential benefits of the arts is central to the discussion and design of effective arts and cultural policies. Further research will help bring clarity and transparency to the debate.

Caron Atlas raises an important point here, one with which centralists, free-marketers and grass-roots advocates can all agree: 'Not calling something a policy does not mean there isn't any. Cultural policies—public and private, implicit and explicit—are made all the time... The challenge is to articulate a clear, pluralistic vision for cultural policymaking that recognises the integral connection between culture, art, and the rest of our lives.'[1]

## Mark Seton asks, 'Will we still be right, mate?

In *The Weekend Australian's Rear View* entitled 'Policy-free zone, please',[2] Imre Salusinszky takes David Throsby's paper to task over the lack of 'solid evidence' for the claims made about cultural impoverishment. He observes: 'These are hardly precise arguments from somebody who calls himself an economist.' But, in support of Professor Throsby, I would argue that this is precisely what he is concerned with addressing. Throsby argues that cultural values are not, ultimately, about measurements but about the sustainability and flourishing of human relationships. His intention is not to offer new measures but to question our present 'cultural' preoccupation with measurement.

Salusinszky also expresses concern about the paper being the first step to determining 'right thinking'. He believes that Throsby's 'soft cultural policy' will merely prolong a 'corruption by groupthink' that Salusinszky believes is responsible for the undermining of the role of the arts in Australia. This seems stereotypically Australian—a kind of 'she'll be right, mate' mentality that believes that if you let things run their natural course, all will be well. But what Throsby reminds us is that people affect other people through their choices and determinations. There is no policy-free zone as Salusinszky would have it. Throsby calls us all to be accountable for the current, often unspoken policies that are being constantly enacted. Furthermore, he invites us to take steps to be transparent and engaged in developing more ethical, equitable and sustainable cultural and social processes. I see in this paper an invitation to mutual accountability.

Throsby relates policy to an ethical thematic that is awkward because it involves accountability for the present and future and some shame over 'unfinished' affairs of the past. These past events lie unreconciled and, it seems, beyond forgiveness, grace and generosity—all things that cannot and should not be measured or figured in by economists. A key attitude that is often evoked to assuage these anxieties is tolerance. Tolerance, as Fiona Jenkins suggests, is finally, a conversation-stopper. I will 'tolerate' you, in public, but, privately, I will continue to resent you, and possibly, undermine you wherever I can. Rather than resorting to tolerance, I believe we will need to draw upon resources from those cultural groups that allow for more sustainable ways of addressing our common vulnerability. A cultural policy entails a duty of care.

## Benjamin Marks on economic fallacies

There may well be elements of 'tall-poppy syndrome' in Australian culture, but there is also something of a 'she'll be right' mentality. A 'she'll be right' policy would be oxymoronic. Yet David Throsby ignores this. He does not propose government disappear to allow Australian culture to flourish, he does not even consider it. For Throsby government could help Australian culture by giving money to the arts through subsidies and protectionist policies. In the following I show why such measures would be counterproductive and unjust.

Throsby begins by trying to define exactly what culture is and ends up being content to equate it with the arts (p. 5). But the arts are also difficult to define, as Paul Costantoura found in his Australia Council study.[3] Having a fuzzy definition is not so bad for most purposes. When talking about legislation, however, it is unacceptable. For if it is claimed that the arts are important for the public good, and we do not know what is art and what is not, then what does the public good amount to? Throsby later defines the 'core creative arts' as 'the production of sound, image and text' (p. 39), which is far too broad a definition for my liking, especially as a basis for legislation.

Throsby claims to be writing in his capacity as an economist (p. 32), but the essay is full of value judgements and economic fallacies. In fact, there are no economic principles displayed in the article at all. He considers government funding of the arts necessary because of the public-goods problem (p. 35). But what if government does something wrong, is that a public-good problem too?

Throsby rehashes the old mercantilist and protectionist fallacies. That tariffs and subsidies 'protect' people from 'villains seeking to impose a homogenised culture on everything and everyone' (p. 28). But at least with businesses this 'homogenisation' can be avoided simply by not buying the product in question. And there is nothing to stop businesses offering a superior product and outdoing the competition. Any attempt by government to give subsidies to benefit one group of entrenched interests or charge tariffs or even ban competitors will mean that the consumer loses out. There will be less incentive to improve their product. It will tend to result in a lower quality service at a higher cost.

On a different matter, John Howard in his many long years in power has done nothing to curb government intervention and distortion of the economy. No matter what you think of Howard he can hardly be called a fan of the market. Yet Throsby claims, 'Howard is an uncompromising advocate of hard-line free-market reform' (p. 18). Throsby is right to say that for the arts to thrive there needs to be a change in government policy. Unfortunately he gets the direction wrong. Not only does Australia not need a cultural policy, we don't want one either.

## Andrew Barnum on mining creativity

The launch of *Platform Papers No.7* (8 February 2006) was incisive and memorable for some key indicators that described very clearly the current climate within the Australian culture and creative economy discourse. The introduction by Cate Blanchett, in some eyes 'the world's greatest actor', gave serious media weight to the event and the plight she has chosen to champion. Her telling of her child's love of the word 'nation', the description of our 'dense and rapid times', of how the repetition of 'how blue the sky is' would cause her to 'tear off my own head' underlined the malaise of an urban population 'living unexamined lives'. She spoke of an environment that needed to become 'proactive versus reactive' and look beyond an arts community currently bound by 'tangible returns'.

Professor Throsby has made a compelling, vital and well-documented appeal for a cultural summit on Australian cultural policy. Its aim would be the 'development of a national cultural policy to protect and affirm [Australian] cultural sovereignty and to promote national unity and an [Australian] identity' (p.3, to adapt a statement from the Canadian Government). A process of creating a national Australian cultural consciousness would seem feasible if it could be successfully promoted to national attention.

Where Throsby is most correct, is in underlining 'a government's' responsibility to foster and generate 'the conditions where creativity, as a key resource', could 'flourish as the core of the creative arts'. A responsibility to promote the conditions for a newly-defined creativity that broadens the existing creative arts model.

In his launch speech Throsby alluded to 'the mine-able potential of our creative resource'. This resonates as a language to pursue if we're to focus and attract the interest of our current political rationalists. For Mr Howard and his colleagues, creativity seems stuck in a hand-out-to-seditious-subversive-artists mindset. He has underlined his party's 'ideological distaste for public sector involvement in any area they see as being better left to private enterprise', remaining 'uncomfortable with the critical and perhaps confrontational stance on sensitive issues that artists and cultural organisations can take'. (p10)

The truth is, the contemporary artist has long revised the notion of a Government-patronised practice and embraced an individually self-sufficient way of sustaining his/her practice. But creative workers *do* expect provision of a framework and vision that recognises and supports their cultural work. This would be the outcome a cultural summit could provide.

A new cultural discourse would require the popular notion of creativity as an 'artists-only playground' to be broadened and redefined as 'the universal process' it has become. Creativity in the so-called new economy needs to be understood as Charles Leadbeater sees it: 'Companies (and individuals) in knowledge-intensive industries compete on the basis of their intangible assets.'[4] Creativity and cultural identity are just such valuable assets. Australia is rich with them. Defining creativity as a type of 'mining intangible assets process' should make sense for economic rationalists looking to get a foothold in these 'dense and rapid times'.

## Raymond Menmuir on seeing ourselves as we are

Professor David Throsby gives a lucid account of government funding of the arts, brief and incomplete though he protests it is. His assessment of the present climate is cogent. It comes as no surprise, therefore, that he thinks it timely and necessary to '… re-examine the directions of our cultural development… how better to discharge our commitments to the arts and explore more openly the cultural foundations of our economic, social and foreign policy?' Plus ça change?

Fifteen years ago when I returned from over 30 years' work abroad, I was asked repeatedly two questions: 'Isn't that blue sky wonderful?' (I had much empathy with Cate Blanchett's mention of blue sky during her opening remarks at the essay's launch) and: 'Isn't it the most beautiful harbour in the world?' Both were phrased rhetorically and yet required an answer. I thought that if either was asked once more I would answer, 'I prefer rain clouds', or, 'It is a toxic cesspool, dangerous to man and fish.'

One further piece of nostalgia: 'It must have been a great culture shock for you—coming back, that is.' I always wondered what they meant by 'culture'. I decided to stand still, as it were, and listen—to the 'white noise', (Cate again). In the very high decibel range was something marked 'funding'; in the high range was 'Australia Council' and variations; and remarkably, the rest of it was recognisable from the 1940s and 50s when I started my career. Plus ça change.

If a re-examination is to be embarked upon, as Throsby pleads, it is vital that we change the way we look at ourselves, that we see what our culture is—now, not what we, for our comfort, think it is or should be, nor conflate culture and 'cultured'. A Lebanese youth said on ABC television last night (9 February) 'I am an Australian. This is my culture. That's the way it is.' He is part of our culture and not only he.

But how is this re-examination to proceed? David Throsby suggests a 'bottom-up' approach, '… whereby grass-roots individuals, communities and others might coalesce around particular issues…'. To recognise that the process of culture is a rising up, not a filtering down one is a salutary step. His suggestion that this may well lead to discussion papers, manifestos, and draft policy statements smacks of the bureaucratic. As a coalface worker, I am inherently suspicious of manifestos and draft policy statements. But if Professor Throsby continues to lend his considerable experience to formalising a cultural policy, coalface workers may well have less reason for concern than they have in the present climate of increasing political interference.

# Gillian McCracken on the need for a cultural policy

This debate must be re-started, and the words have to be found to argue why a national cultural policy is fundamental to Australian society. Throsby raises a number of important issues and many of us share his unease. Some of these might be resolved with a change of government. However the current Opposition gives me little confidence—it has shown scant commitment to a vision and values different from those of the Government. Prime Minister Keating's *Creative Nation* was a fundamentally good idea with flaws. Although it was signed off in Cabinet, *Creative Nation* had few committed advocates once Keating was gone. The Opposition has not raised it as an issue, never mind a policy, since that time.

What is culture and what would a cultural policy provide? A cultural policy must have Federal Government acceptance but it should not be a blueprint for changing Australian society. The fundamentals must be embedded within Australian society as it is, rather than what a few want it to be. Each individual needs to feel that their own histories and lives have contributed to the essence of the policy and that it is meant to have cultural benefit for all Australians. Our media is the obvious vehicle to carry some of this debate and in particular TV and radio. More resources for our internationally recognised writers, directors, and technicians to produce challenging drama for Australian TV would be a start.

Sebastian Smee in his article on biennales[5] exposes the dilemma of creating an environment of support for contemporary art. How do you establish a cultural policy that allows for chaos, dissent and government discomfort and at the same time supports infrastructure to underpin arts activities? Many local Councils have followed government directives developing 'cultural plans' that include art programs and public art. Is this adequate? Such plans should be grounded on a sound philosophical base flowing from a well-researched national cultural policy that includes the arts and also attitudes and aspirations that enrich people's lives.

Fundamental to my research for a Masters degree was the premise that the art made in a society contribute to an understanding of what makes each society specific. With the assistance of two Ngarrindjeri women I learned about the intricate cultural uniqueness of these people through their practice of basketry. This practice developed as a direct response to their geographic location, flora and source of food. It provided a process for every practical aspect of their lives from birth to death, for sharing stories and for passing down history, and it provided a metaphorical narrative for the gradual evolution of their culture. Could this practice be extrapolated to current society? I am adamant that it can.

Many art practices sustain and reinforce the reality that many different cultural voices weave together to be contemporary Australia. I am grateful to David Throsby for re-kindling the debate. I hope it doesn't follow down the same paths as previous debates which have locked it into partisan politics.

## Catherine Baldwin on the benefits of art

Some people may struggle with the notion of culture representing anything beyond the easily recognised arts and heritage experiences. However, quite clearly our culture is not only our experience of the performing, visual and museum arts which Throsby places at the 'core', but is defined by our values, beliefs, interactions and how we think of ourselves.

The role of government is critical in providing leadership and support. Without government intervention, there would still be artists and art works, and people would congregate to share their personal and collective experiences. However, as Throsby points out, there is a great deal to be gained, including economic gains, from the sponsoring of a vibrant, relevant, interactive and creative environment. Whether it's nurturing the creativity of school children or CSIRO scientists, Australia has a deal to gain from the innovation for which we have become renowned.

We already have a de facto cultural policy if you review the cumulative effect of the many decisions made by government on behalf of the community in areas such as: our international and racial relationships, our enthusiasm for sport, our attitude to the natural environment, our view of indigenous people, our telecommunications and media industry. What David Throsby and others are calling for is a focused discussion about the way we want to see ourselves and be seen by others—this might have been facilitated through support for the UNESCO cultural declaration.

Financial assistance to the arts could be more generous, whether from governments or corporates, and would have the benefit of allowing greater risk-taking by artists and by the communities they serve. We rely on our arts community to reflect our lives, to enable us to re-examine ourselves, to understand ethnic diversity, to appreciate beauty and express our individual and collective creativity. Putting an economic framework around the value of culture to a community can get people talking and thinking, but it will take vision from our leaders, and an understanding of the issues by the public, to really make a difference.

1.  Caron Atlas, *Cultural Policy: What is it? Who makes it? Why does it matter?* (New York Foundation for the Arts)

www.nyfa.org/files_uploaded/Pages_65-68.pdf

2    Imre Salusinszky, 'Policy-free zone, please', *Weekend Australian*, 11–12 February 2006.

3    Paul Costantoura, *Australians and the Arts* (Sydney: Federation Press, 2001)

4    Charles Leadbeater, *Living on thin air: the new economy.* (London: Penguin 1999)

5.   Imre Salusinszky, 'Policy-free zone, please', *Weekend Australian*, 11–12 February 2006.

## Backlist: the debates continue

No. 1: 'Our ABC' a Dying Culture? One Way Forward in Arts Programming

MARTIN HARRISON's seminal essay on the decline in ABC arts production and commentary.

ISBN 0 9581212 4 9     RRP $12.95

No. 2: Survival of the Fittest: The Artist versus the Corporate World

CHRISTOPHER LATHAM applauds the ingenuity of independent artists in a time of rapid technological advance.

ISBN 0 9581213 6 2     RRP $12.95

No. 3: Trapped by the Past: Why Our Theatre is Facing Paralysis

JULIAN MEYRICK assaults the 'middle-aged' structure of the performing arts and calls for change.

ISBN 0 9581213 7 0     RRP $12.95

No. 4: The Myth of the Mainstream: Politics and the Performing Arts in Australia

ROBYN ARCHER outlines how and why we have sold out the arts to populism.

ISBN 0 9757301 0 X     RRP $12.95

No. 5: Shooting Through: Australian Film and the Brain Drain

STORRY WALTON asserts our filmmakers are an unrecognised asset waiting to be realised.

ISBN 09757301 1 8     RRP $12.95

No. 6: Art in a Cold Climate: Rethinking the Australia Council

KEITH GALLASCH argues that the loss of the New Media and Community Development boards has damaged innovation.

ISBN 09753 012 6     RRP 12.95

**No. 7: Does Australia Need a Cultural Policy?**

DAVID THROSBY on the values that bind us together.

ISBN 0 9757 013 4     RRP $13.95

# Subscribe to **Platform Papers**

Individual recommended retail price: $13.95

**HAVE THE PAPERS DELIVERED QUARTERLY TO YOUR DOOR**

**4 issues for $55.00 including postage within Australia**

**SPECIAL OFFER: *Currency Companion to Music and Dance***

**Subscribe to *Platform Papers* and purchase a copy of the *Currency Companion to Music and Dance* (valued at $89.95) for $30.00 (including postage)**

'*A major reference work which lays out the colourful tapestry of Australian music and dance cultures with such thoroughness and breadth of vision*' **Paul Grabowsky**, composer

704 pp, 370 entries, 15 000 index entries

___ I would like to subscribe to 4 issues of *Platform Papers* for $55.00

___ I would like to subscribe to 4 issues of *Platform Papers* plus purchase a copy of the *Currency Companion to Music and Dance* for a total of $85.00

I would like my subscription to start from: ___ this issue

___ the next issue

Name_____

Address_____

_____

_____ State _____ Postcode _____

Email _____

Telephone _____

Please make cheques payable to Currency House Inc.

Or charge: ___ Mastercard ___ Bankcard ___ Visa

Card no. ___ ___ ___ ___ ___ ___ ___ ___ ___ ___ ___ ___

___ ___ ___ ___ Expiry date _____ Signature _____

Fax this form to Currency House Inc. at: 02 9319 3649

Or post to: Currency House Inc., PO Box 2270, Strawberry Hills NSW 2012 Australia

CURRENCY HOUSE